No Carbs No Sugar

A Weight Loss Guide for Women with Easy, Delicious Recipes and a 7-Day Meal Plan

mf

copyright © 2025 Mary Golanna

All rights reserved No part of this book may be reproduced, or stored in a retrieval system, or transmitted in any form or by any means, electronic, mechanical, photocopying, recording, or otherwise, without express written permission of the publisher.

Disclaimer

By reading this disclaimer, you are accepting the terms of the disclaimer in full. If you disagree with this disclaimer, please do not read the guide.

All of the content within this guide is provided for informational and educational purposes only, and should not be accepted as independent medical or other professional advice. The author is not a doctor, physician, nurse, mental health provider, or registered nutritionist/dietician. Therefore, using and reading this guide does not establish any form of a physician-patient relationship.

Always consult with a physician or another qualified health provider with any issues or questions you might have regarding any sort of medical condition. Do not ever disregard any qualified professional medical advice or delay seeking that advice because of anything you have read in this guide. The information in this guide is not intended to be any sort of medical advice and should not be used in lieu of any medical advice by a licensed and qualified medical professional.

The information in this guide has been compiled from a variety of known sources. However, the author cannot attest to or guarantee the accuracy of each source and thus should not be held liable for any errors or omissions.

You acknowledge that the publisher of this guide will not be held liable for any loss or damage of any kind incurred as a result of this guide or the reliance on any information provided within this guide. You acknowledge and agree that you assume all risk and responsibility for any action you undertake in response to the information in this guide.

Using this guide does not guarantee any particular result (e.g., weight loss or a cure). By reading this guide, you acknowledge that there are no guarantees to any specific outcome or results you can expect.

All product names, diet plans, or names used in this guide are for identification purposes only and are the property of their respective owners. The use of these names does not imply endorsement. All other trademarks cited herein are the property of their respective owners.

Where applicable, this guide is not intended to be a substitute for the original work of this diet plan and is, at most, a supplement to the original work for this diet plan and never a direct substitute. This guide is a personal expression of the facts of that diet plan.

Where applicable, persons shown in the cover images are stock photography models and the publisher has obtained the rights to use the images through license agreements with third-party stock image companies.

Table of Contents

Introduction — 7
Why No Carbs and No Sugar? — 9
    Understanding Carbohydrates and Sugars — 9
    The Role of Carbs and Sugar in Weight Gain — 10
    The Benefits of Eliminating Carbs and Sugar — 12
How Carbs and Sugar Impact the Body — 13
    Physical Impact — 13
    Hormonal Imbalance — 14
Women's Unique Weight-Loss Challenges — 18
    Metabolic Differences Between Men and Women — 18
    The Role of Hormones — 19
    Common Obstacles Women Face — 20
Use Cases for No-Carb and No-Sugar Diet in Women — 25
    Diabetes Management — 25
    Weight Loss Strategies for Obesity — 26
    Managing Polycystic Ovary Syndrome (PCOS) — 26
    Treatment of Epilepsy in Women — 27
    Support for Non-Alcoholic Fatty Liver Disease (NAFLD) — 27
    Cancer Patient Dietary Protocols — 27
    Management of Chronic Candida Overgrowth — 28
    Autoimmune Nutritional Protocols — 28
How Does a No-Carb and No-Sugar Diet Work in the Body? — 29
    Shifting to Fat as Fuel — 29
    Stabilizing Insulin Levels — 30
    Supporting Metabolic Health — 31
    Who Benefits Most? — 32
5 Step-by-Guide to Starting a No-Carb, No-Sugar Diet for Busy Women — 33
    Step 1: Set Clear Goals and Prep Your Mindset — 33

    Step 2: Clean Out Your Pantry and Restock Smartly   37
    Step 3: Make Smart Grocery Choices   42
    Step 4: Track Your Progress   47
    Step 5: Reach Out for Support   48
    Foods to Eat in a No-Carb, No-Sugar Diet   49
    Foods to Avoid in a No-Carb, No-Sugar Diet   53

7-Day No Carbs and No Sugar Meal Plan   59
    Day 1   59
    Day 2   60
    Day 3   61
    Day 4   62
    Day 5   63
    Day 6   63
    Day 7   64

Sample Recipes   66
    Spinach & Cheese Omelette Recipe   67
    Grilled Lemon Herb Chicken with Sautéed Zucchini   69
    Avocado Egg Cups Recipe   71
    Grilled Steak Salad   73
    Scrambled Eggs with Turkey Sausage   75
    Turkey Lettuce Wraps   76
    Grilled Chicken Thighs with Steamed Cauliflower Rice   78
    Vegetable Frittata   79
    Grilled Trout with Roasted Brussels Sprouts   81
    Zucchini Noodles with Pesto Shrimp   83
    Poached Eggs with Sliced Avocado   84
    Herb-Roasted Chicken with Spinach Salad   85
    Pan-Seared Cod with Sautéed Kale   87

Conclusion   89
FAQs   92
References and Helpful Links   95

Introduction

Losing weight can feel impossible when juggling the demands of a career, family, and everything else life throws your way. Between hectic schedules and endless responsibilities, finding the time and energy to focus on healthier eating can seem out of reach. Add in conflicting diet advice, and the whole process becomes frustrating and overwhelming. But achieving weight-loss goals doesn't have to mean complicating an already busy routine.

With an emphasis on simplicity and flexibility, this approach helps busy women adopt a no-carbs, no-sugar diet for effective weight loss. It's about creating a plan that fits seamlessly into a packed lifestyle, without rigid rules or unrealistic restrictions. It encourages progress over perfection and redefines what healthy living can look like in the midst of daily chaos.

In this guide, we will talk about the following:

- Why No Carbs and No Sugar?
- How Carbs and Sugar Impact the Body
- Women's Unique Weight-Loss Challenges

- Use Cases for No-Carb and No-Sugar Diet in Women
- How Does a No-Carb and No-Sugar Diet Work in the Body?
- 5 Step-by-Guide to Starting a No-Carb, No-Sugar Diet for Busy Women
- 7-Day No Carbs and No Sugar Meal Plan
- Sample Recipes

The goal is to empower women to take control of their health with small, manageable steps that make a big difference over time. Instead of focusing on quick fixes, the purpose is to inspire sustainable habits that build confidence and deliver results. Each piece of advice is rooted in the reality of balancing personal goals with life's many demands. It's about making weight loss feel achievable, even with a full plate.

Keep reading to discover how a no-carbs, no-sugar diet can fit into your busy lifestyle and help you achieve your weight loss goals without feeling overwhelmed. Whether you're a working mom, a student, or someone with a hectic schedule, this approach can be tailored to fit your unique needs and make healthy eating a more manageable part of your daily routine.

By the end of this guide, you'll have a better understanding of the benefits of a no-carbs, no-sugar diet and how it can positively impact your overall health. You'll also have practical tips and strategies to implement this lifestyle change in a sustainable way.

Why No Carbs and No Sugar?

Understanding why carbohydrates and sugars are removed from a diet is crucial for those looking to make serious changes. By breaking down what they are, how they interact with the body, and the potential benefits of cutting them, this chapter provides the foundation for a healthier lifestyle.

Understanding Carbohydrates and Sugars

Carbohydrates and sugars are essential components of many foods, but they aren't all created the same. Carbohydrates, often called "carbs," are macronutrients that your body uses for energy. They can be broken into two main types — simple and complex.

- ***Simple Carbohydrates*** consist of sugar molecules that are quickly broken down by the body. They're commonly found in foods like candy, white bread, soda, and pastries. These cause rapid spikes in blood sugar, followed by a crash that leaves people feeling tired and craving more sugar.
- ***Complex Carbohydrates***, on the other hand, are made up of longer chains of sugar molecules and take more

time to digest. Foods like whole grains and starchy vegetables fall into this category. While they're often deemed healthier, they still turn into sugar once metabolized.

When it comes to sugar itself, there's another layer to consider.

- *Natural Sugars* are found in whole fruits, dairy, and some vegetables. They're packaged with fiber, vitamins, and minerals, which slow down digestion and help regulate blood sugar levels.
- *Added Sugars* are what food manufacturers sneak into processed foods, from sauces to snacks, for a hit of sweetness. These are the culprits that can quietly derail a diet. High fructose corn syrup, cane sugar, and syrups are common examples.

Breaking down these distinctions shows that not all carbs are inherently bad, but certain types can have disproportionately negative effects on the body.

The Role of Carbs and Sugar in Weight Gain

To understand weight gain, it's crucial to examine how carbohydrates and sugars are metabolized in the body. When carbs are consumed, they're broken down into glucose — the body's primary energy source. Glucose enters the bloodstream, signaling the pancreas to release insulin, a hormone that helps cells absorb sugar and store any excess in the liver or as fat.

Now, here's where the problem lies.

- ***Insulin Spikes and Fat Storage***: If someone eats a meal rich in simple carbs, the flood of glucose into the bloodstream leads to a massive insulin spike. While this helps clear glucose from the blood quickly, it can also cause the body to prioritize fat storage. The liver converts any surplus glucose into fat, which then settles in areas like the abdomen, thighs, or hips.
- ***Cravings and Overeating***: The aftermath of an insulin spike isn't pretty. Shortly after clearing out all that sugar, blood sugar levels drop dramatically, leaving the person feeling sluggish and hungry again. This leads to a cycle of overeating, as the body signals for quick, accessible energy—which usually means reaching for more carbs or sugary snacks.

Consider this example. Someone eats a muffin for breakfast—seemingly innocent enough. While it provides a quick hit of energy, it sets off an insulin response. By mid-morning, their blood sugar has plummeted, triggering a trip to the vending machine for a candy bar. The body is caught in a vicious loop of high sugar intake, fat storage, and persistent hunger.

The Benefits of Eliminating Carbs and Sugar

Taking carbs and sugar out of the equation interrupts this cycle and brings a series of positive changes.

1. *Steady Energy Levels*: Without blood sugar spikes and crashes, energy stays consistent throughout the day. Fat and protein provide longer-lasting fuel, so no more afternoon slumps or coffee runs.
2. *Fewer Cravings*: Cutting out insulin-spiking foods reduces cravings, especially for sugary snacks. Over time, your palate adapts, making it easier to resist sweets and carb-heavy foods.
3. *Boosted Fat-Burning*: Eating fewer carbs shifts the body to burn fat for energy, a process called ketosis. This helps use stored fat more effectively and lowers insulin levels.
4. *Improved Metabolism*: Reducing carbs and sugar lowers the risk of insulin resistance and improves overall health, from hormonal balance to reduced inflammation.

Understanding these dynamics shows why a no-carb, no-sugar diet plan isn't a passing trend but a functional approach to health and weight management. By focusing on foods that fuel the body naturally, busy women can regain control over their energy, appetite, and long-term wellness.

How Carbs and Sugar Impact the Body

Understanding the effects of carbohydrates and sugars on the body goes beyond simply seeing their role in weight gain. These substances influence physical health, hormone balance, and even mental well-being. Examining these impacts provides a clear insight into why reducing carb and sugar intake is a constructive step for many women.

Physical Impact

Carbs and sugar play a direct role in the regulation of energy levels and metabolic health. When they're consumed excessively, the consequences can wreak havoc on the body.

1. **Blood Sugar Spikes and Crashes**

   When sugary or carb-heavy foods are eaten, blood sugar levels rise rapidly. This triggers the pancreas to flood the body with insulin to clear glucose from the bloodstream. While this keeps blood sugar from remaining dangerously high, it often overcompensates, causing blood sugar to drop dramatically — a crash.

People experience these drops as fatigue, irritability, or even hunger soon after eating.

This rollercoaster effect on blood sugar not only creates a cycle of constant snacking but also wears out the body's insulin response mechanisms.

2. Risk of Insulin Resistance and Type 2 Diabetes

When high-carb and sugary diets persist, cells become less responsive to insulin — a condition called insulin resistance. This forces the pancreas to produce even more insulin to keep blood sugar in check, ultimately straining the system.

Left unmanaged, insulin resistance can lead to Type 2 diabetes, a chronic condition that increases the risk for heart disease, nerve damage, kidney issues, and other serious health complications. This progression highlights how significant the long-term effects of these dietary choices can be.

Hormonal Imbalance

Particularly for women, carbs and sugar can disrupt hormonal balance, which impacts not just weight loss but also energy, mood, and even reproductive health.

1. **Effects on Cortisol and Stress**

   High-sugar diets elevate cortisol, the body's primary stress hormone. Over time, elevated cortisol levels can lead to fat storage, particularly in the abdominal area, and contribute to feelings of stress and anxiety. While sugar may initially feel like a comfort food during stressful times, it exacerbates the physiological stress response.

2. **The Relationship Between Sugar, Carbs, and Estrogen/Progesterone Imbalance**

   Carbs and sugars can also disturb the delicate balance of estrogen and progesterone in women's bodies. High-carb diets have been linked to increased levels of estrogen, which can exacerbate hormone-related issues like premenstrual syndrome (PMS) or polycystic ovary syndrome (PCOS).

   Additionally, insulin resistance can interfere with overall hormone regulation, potentially impacting ovulation and fertility. Cutting back on carbs and sugar allows these systems to stabilize, promoting better hormonal health.

3. **Mental Health Effects**

   What many don't realize is how strongly diet influences mental well-being. Carbs and sugar affect the brain in ways that can lead to long-term cognitive and emotional challenges.

4. Carb Addiction and Its Similarity to Drug Addiction

Sugar and simple carbs act like addictive substances, triggering the brain's reward center to release dopamine. Over time, this creates cravings, as the brain demands more to feel the same pleasure. This cycle of overconsumption mimics drug addiction, leading to unhealthy eating habits. Cutting back on sugar and carbs can break this pattern and promote a healthier relationship with food.

5. Link Between Sugar and Mood Swings, Brain Fog, and Fatigue

The ups and downs in blood sugar caused by carbs and sugar don't just affect energy—they also impact mood. Spikes can cause irritability, while crashes may lead to fatigue or sadness.

Overindulging can also harm focus, leading to brain fog or difficulty concentrating. Many women report sharper focus and steadier moods when they cut back on sugar and carb-heavy foods, highlighting the benefits of these changes.

Understanding how carbs and sugar affect physical health, hormones, and mental well-being helps women make better choices. These substances don't just affect weight—they influence overall quality of life. For busy women, this knowledge can be a key step toward reclaiming energy, balance, and clarity.

Women's Unique Weight-Loss Challenges

When it comes to weight loss, women face unique biological and hormonal factors that can make the process more challenging compared to men. Understanding these differences can help women approach weight loss with realistic expectations and strategies tailored to their individual needs.

Metabolic Differences Between Men and Women

One key difference lies in the way women's bodies naturally store and use fat. From an evolutionary perspective, women are biologically predisposed to store more fat than men. This stems from the vital role fat plays in reproductive health. Fat stores provide essential energy reserves needed during pregnancy and breastfeeding, making them a survival mechanism for women's bodies.

Men, on the other hand, generally have more muscle mass, which increases their resting metabolic rate (the rate at which their bodies burn calories at rest). Muscle tissue burns more calories than fat tissue, so even when inactive, men tend to burn more energy. For women, the higher proportion of fat and lower muscle mass means they burn fewer calories than men, making weight loss a slower process.

The Role of Hormones

Hormones also play a pivotal role in women's weight-loss challenges, particularly estrogen and progesterone. These hormones fluctuate throughout a woman's life, particularly during menstrual cycles, pregnancy, and menopause, and they influence how fat is stored and metabolized.

- *Estrogen and Fat Storage*: Estrogen encourages fat storage in the hips, thighs, and buttocks as part of the body's preparation for childbearing. While normal and healthy, this can make losing fat in these areas more difficult for women.
- *Estrogen's Impact on Metabolism*: During perimenopause and menopause, declining estrogen slows metabolism, leading to weight gain, especially around the abdomen. Many women notice weight gain during this stage, even without changes in diet or activity.
- *The Role of Progesterone*: Progesterone can cause water retention and bloating, making women feel heavier during the luteal phase of their cycle. While it

doesn't cause fat gain, it can still be frustrating and affect motivation.
- ***Hormonal Shifts and Cravings***: Fluctuations in estrogen and progesterone during the menstrual cycle can trigger cravings for sugary or high-carb foods, which may derail weight-loss efforts if not managed.

Understanding biological and hormonal differences isn't about excuses—it's about setting realistic expectations and being kind to yourself during weight loss. Women's bodies are built to store fat and respond to hormonal changes, which can make losing weight harder.

By acknowledging these challenges, women can focus on strategies that work with their bodies, like strength training to build muscle, managing stress to control cortisol, and prioritizing balanced nutrition.

Most importantly, women should approach weight loss with patience, persistence, and a tailored plan. While it may take longer than for men, understanding these factors can lead to healthier, lasting results.

Common Obstacles Women Face

Women often encounter unique barriers on their weight-loss journeys, stemming from biological, emotional, and lifestyle factors. By understanding these challenges more deeply, women can develop strategies that work within their realities, not against them.

Emotional Eating and Hormonal Changes

Hormonal fluctuations throughout a woman's life can strongly influence mood, hunger, and cravings, often leading to emotional eating.

- *Menstrual Cycle*: During the luteal phase (after ovulation and before a period), progesterone rises, and estrogen drops. This hormonal shift can cause fatigue, irritability, and cravings for comfort foods like sweets or carbs. Emotional eating is common during this time as women may seek temporary relief through food.
- *Pregnancy*: Pregnancy causes major hormonal changes along with physical and emotional demands. Higher levels of hormones like hCG and progesterone can lead to nausea, cravings, or appetite changes. These shifts, while natural, can make it harder to eat a balanced diet, leading some women to overeat or choose less nutritious foods.
- *Menopause*: Menopause introduces lower estrogen levels, which can disrupt sleep, affect mood, and slow metabolism. These changes are often coupled with stress or feelings of frustration about weight gain, which can drive emotional eating as a coping mechanism.

How to Manage Emotional Eating:

- Recognize patterns and triggers, such as certain phases in your cycle or moments of stress. Keeping a journal can help identify recurring themes.
- Have healthier comfort options readily available, like dark chocolate, yogurt with fresh fruit, or a handful of nuts, to satisfy cravings without overindulging.
- Practice mindfulness during meals by eating slowly and listening to hunger signals rather than eating out of habit or emotion.

Stress and Weight

Stress is another major barrier to weight loss, both physically and emotionally. When stress levels are high, the body releases cortisol, a hormone that helps regulate the stress response.

- *Cortisol and Fat Storage*: Chronic stress keeps cortisol levels elevated, which can signal the body to store fat, particularly around the midsection. This survival mechanism was essential in times when food was scarce, but in today's world, it often leads to unwanted weight gain.
- *Cortisol and Hunger*: Cortisol also influences hunger hormones, like ghrelin and leptin. When cortisol rises, ghrelin (the "hunger hormone") increases while leptin (the hormone that tells you you're full) decreases. This

imbalance can make you feel hungrier and less satisfied, even after eating a meal.

How to Combat Stress:

- Incorporate stress management techniques into your daily routine, such as yoga, meditation, or deep-breathing exercises.
- Exercise regularly, as it not only helps burn calories but also reduces cortisol levels and improves mood.
- Ensure you get enough sleep, as inadequate rest can amplify cortisol production and increase cravings for unhealthy foods.

Time Constraints

For many women, time feels like their biggest obstacle when trying to achieve weight-loss goals. Between work, family commitments, social obligations, and personal downtime, it can be difficult to carve out time for meal planning or exercise.

- *Meal Planning Struggles*: Preparing healthy meals requires time for grocery shopping, cooking, and cleaning up—all tasks that can feel overwhelming, particularly during busy weeks. This can lead many women to rely on fast food or processed meals, which are often high in sugars and unhealthy fats.
- *Lack of Time for Exercise*: Regular physical activity is essential for weight loss, but finding even 30

minutes a day for a workout can feel impossible when juggling full schedules.

Time-Saving Strategies:

- *Meal Prep in Advance*: Set aside a block of time each week, like Sunday afternoon, to plan and prepare meals. Chop vegetables, cook proteins in bulk, or portion out snacks to save time during the week.
- *Opt for Mini Workouts*: If you can't find time for a full 30- or 60-minute workout, break it into smaller chunks. Even 10- to 15-minute sessions of walking, stretching, or strength training throughout the day can accumulate into meaningful exercise.
- *Double-Duty Activities*: Look for ways to pair exercise with other tasks. For example, take the kids to the park and join them for active play, or do bodyweight exercises while watching your favorite show.

By tackling emotional eating, stress, and time constraints with small, practical steps, women can create a more sustainable and empowering path toward weight loss. Remember, progress is more important than perfection—every little effort towards better health adds up over time.

Use Cases for No-Carb and No-Sugar Diet in Women

The no-carb and no-sugar diet offers a versatile approach for women, with targeted applications ranging from managing chronic health conditions to supporting weight loss goals, all requiring careful personalization and professional guidance to ensure safety and effectiveness.

Diabetes Management

A no-carb, no-sugar diet can be applied as a strict method to regulate blood sugar levels in women with diabetes, particularly Type 2. By cutting out carbohydrates and sugars, which have a direct impact on blood glucose, women might simplify blood sugar management.

Under medical supervision, this dietary approach could be used alongside medication to support glucose consistency. Women adopting this diet must monitor their blood sugar frequently and may need adjustments in their insulin or other diabetes medications based on how the body responds to the restricted intake.

Weight Loss Strategies for Obesity

This approach is sometimes used by women aiming to lose weight when traditional calorie-restricted diets have not worked. It involves completely removing carbohydrate and sugar sources to focus on proteins and fats, which can lead to fewer cravings and controlled appetite.

Though demanding and restrictive, this diet is implemented under strict supervision as an intervention to break specific eating patterns or reset dietary habits that perpetuate excess calorie consumption.

Managing Polycystic Ovary Syndrome (PCOS)

Women with PCOS who experience insulin resistance often turn to low-carb diets, but in extreme or well-targeted contexts, a no-carb, no-sugar diet may also be used. This stricter nutritional framework is applied to address hormonal fluctuations and help improve insulin sensitivity.

For women with PCOS, this diet might also support managing the frequent cycles of hunger caused by unstable blood sugar levels. Such a dietary application would typically be combined with regular monitoring and collaboration with an endocrinologist or dietitian.

Treatment of Epilepsy in Women

The no-carb, no-sugar diet can serve as a basis for the medical ketogenic diet, which is highly effective in controlling seizures in some forms of epilepsy. Women with this condition may use this diet plan under strict medical guidelines if other treatments are not effective. Notably, every detail of nutrient intake is carefully calculated to maintain a ketogenic state, as even small deviations could reduce the diet's efficacy for seizure control.

Support for Non-Alcoholic Fatty Liver Disease (NAFLD)

For women diagnosed with NAFLD, a no-carb and no-sugar eating plan can be applied to reduce the liver's exposure to excess sugars and carbohydrates, which contribute to fat storage in the organ. This dietary application is often guided by hepatologists or dietitians to ensure it aligns with overall liver health goals while avoiding nutrient deficiencies.

Cancer Patient Dietary Protocols

Some cancer treatments or therapeutic approaches involve no-sugar diets to limit the potential "fuel" for rapidly dividing cancer cells. Women undergoing treatment may follow a no-carb, no-sugar diet under the supervision of an oncologist and nutritionist as part of a broader treatment protocol. This use case is experimental in some areas but is closely monitored as an adjunct therapy.

Management of Chronic Candida Overgrowth

A no-carb, no-sugar diet is sometimes applied to address chronic Candida infections in women. By removing sugars and carbs that feed yeast in the body, this diet is used as part of a protocol to balance gut microbiota. It often accompanies antifungal treatments to ensure a holistic approach to resolving the issue.

Autoimmune Nutritional Protocols

For women with autoimmune conditions such as Hashimoto's thyroiditis, a no-carb, no-sugar diet may be part of an elimination or reset phase in specific dietary protocols. This approach is applied to uncover food triggers, reduce inflammation, and identify dietary sensitivities that worsen the autoimmune response.

These use cases must be tailored to individual needs and monitored by healthcare professionals to ensure safety and effectiveness.

How Does a No-Carb and No-Sugar Diet Work in the Body?

A no-carb and no-sugar diet creates significant physiological changes that shift how your body functions, ultimately promoting fat loss and stabilizing energy levels. By cutting out carbs and sugars, you encourage your body to use fat as its primary energy source, while also minimizing blood sugar spikes and insulin fluctuations. Here's a closer look at how it works and why it can be so effective.

Shifting to Fat as Fuel

Carbohydrates are typically the body's go-to energy source. When you eat carbs, they are broken down into glucose (sugar), which enters the bloodstream and provides fuel for your cells. However, when carbs and sugars are no longer part of your diet, your body has to find an alternative energy source—this is where fat comes into play.

- *Ketosis*: On a no-carb and no-sugar diet, your body enters a metabolic state called ketosis. With no carbohydrates to burn, your liver starts breaking down fat into molecules called ketones, which become your new energy source. Ketones are incredibly efficient, providing steady energy without the roller-coaster effects of sugar highs and crashes.

- ***Fat Burning and Weight Loss***: By relying on fat for fuel, your body starts tapping into its fat stores more effectively. This can lead to significant weight loss, especially when combined with a caloric deficit. Burning fat instead of glucose not only reduces stored fat but also prevents your body from making new fat deposits.

Stabilizing Insulin Levels

When you eat carbs and sugar, your blood sugar rises, triggering your body to release insulin. Insulin's job is to help your cells absorb glucose for energy, but it also tells your body to store excess glucose as fat.

- ***Reducing Insulin Spikes***: By eliminating carbs and sugar, you keep blood sugar levels stable, which means your body produces less insulin. With fewer insulin spikes, your body enters a more stable, fat-burning mode, instead of constantly storing fat.
- ***Improving Insulin Sensitivity***: Over time, a no-carb and no-sugar diet can improve insulin sensitivity. This means your body becomes better at processing blood

sugar, reducing the risk of insulin resistance and conditions like Type 2 diabetes.

Supporting Metabolic Health

A no-carb and no-sugar diet doesn't just help you lose weight—it can also enhance overall metabolic health by addressing key factors like blood sugar stability, inflammation, and appetite control.

- *Reduced Cravings*: Without the constant blood sugar fluctuations caused by sugar and refined carbs, cravings naturally decrease. Instead of dealing with hunger pangs every few hours, you'll likely feel full for longer, as fat and protein provide more lasting satiety.
- *Lowering Inflammation*: High-sugar diets are linked to increased levels of inflammation in the body, which can contribute to chronic conditions like heart disease, arthritis, and obesity. Cutting out sugar and carbs can reduce inflammation, leading to improvements in overall health and well-being.
- *Boosting Energy*: Both physical and mental energy levels stabilize on this diet. Without sugar crashes, you're likely to experience consistent energy throughout the day, along with improved focus and mental clarity.

Who Benefits Most?

This diet works particularly well for individuals who struggle with weight loss, blood sugar issues, or inflammation. It's especially effective for women dealing with hormonal imbalances or insulin resistance, as it helps regulate hormones like insulin and cortisol while promoting fat loss.

By eliminating carbs and sugar, you create a metabolic environment that prioritizes fat burning and reduces fat storage. While it takes an adjustment period to adapt to this way of eating, the long-term benefits—like stabilized energy levels, reduced cravings, and enhanced metabolic health—make it a powerful approach for those looking to improve their weight and overall well-being.

5 Step-by-Guide to Starting a No-Carb, No-Sugar Diet for Busy Women

If you're looking to boost your energy, shed extra weight, and feel more in control of your health, a no-carb, no-sugar diet can be a game-changer. For busy women like you, though, sticking to a new eating plan can feel daunting—especially with a packed schedule and endless responsibilities. But don't worry! With the right strategies, you can make this transition easier and more sustainable. Here's a step-by-step guide to help you get started:

Step 1: Set Clear Goals and Prep Your Mindset

Starting a no-carb, no-sugar diet is a major lifestyle shift, so understanding why you're making this change is the foundation for your success. This step isn't just about deciding to change your eating habits—it's about anchoring yourself to meaningful and motivating reasons that will keep you going when temptations arise or when the adjustment feels tough. Here's how to set yourself up for success:

Understand the Importance of Setting Goals

When you're busy, it's easy to lose focus on why you started something new. Setting clear goals gives you a sense of purpose and focus. Goals help you move forward with intention rather than feeling overwhelmed or aimless.

Whether those goals are weight loss, improved energy, better skin, or simply feeling in control of your diet, make them personal to you. The clearer your goals are, the more they'll energize and motivate you.

Example Goals for Inspiration:

- "I want to lose 10 pounds within two months so I feel confident and healthy for vacation."
- "I want to boost my energy and focus, so my weekday productivity doesn't dip during the afternoon lull."
- "I want to reduce my sugar cravings to feel more in control of my food choices."

How to Effectively Set Goals

Take time to be specific about what you want to achieve and why it matters. Write your goals down in a journal, post them on a sticky note near your bathroom mirror, or set up a daily reminder on your phone. Make your goals realistic but inspiring—something you're eager to work toward but not so extreme that it feels intimidating.

Consider breaking them into small, actionable milestones. For example, instead of "completely cutting sugar in a week," aim to "go 48 hours without sugar this week" as a starting point.

Practical Tip: Use the SMART framework for your goals—make them Specific, Measurable, Attainable, Relevant, and Time-bound.

Visual Reminders to Stay Motivated

Keeping your goals visible is critical. Busy schedules can pull your focus in a dozen directions, but constant visual reminders will nudge you toward your commitment.

- Create a vision board with images of healthy meals, inspiring quotes, or something that symbolizes your "why."
- Use sticky notes on your fridge or pantry with encouraging reminders like "You're choosing health over habits!"
- Schedule reminders on your phone to pop up at meal times with affirmations like "This is fueling my best self!"

Shift Your Mindset for the Journey

Acknowledging that cutting carbs and sugar will feel tough at first can help you stay kind to yourself during this transition. Sugar, in particular, is addictive, and cravings or even withdrawal symptoms are common as your body adjusts. Remind yourself that this discomfort is temporary, and the benefits will outweigh the short-term challenges.

Focus on what you're gaining rather than what you think you're missing. Instead of, "I can't have desserts," say, "I'm fueling my body with nourishing foods that make me feel amazing." A positive mindset not only makes the process more sustainable but also lowers the stress that often derails dietary changes.

Daily Affirmations to Keep You Grounded

Affirmations are a simple yet powerful way to boost your confidence and keep your commitment alive. Start your morning by repeating a few aloud or writing them in your journal. These statements can help train your brain to focus on the positives of your new lifestyle.

- "I choose foods that energize me."
- "Every meal is a step closer to my goal."
- "Challenging myself today sets me up for success tomorrow."

To go further, combine these affirmations with visualization techniques. Picture yourself thriving on your new diet—full of energy, wearing your favorite outfit, or enjoying your improved focus and mood.

Remember, no-carb, no-sugar isn't just about food. It's about making a choice to prioritize your health and success. There will be days when it feels easier and others when the effort feels harder, but sticking to your goals will build resilience and strength. Lean into the process with enthusiasm and self-compassion. You're not just creating a new diet—you're cultivating a healthier, stronger you.

Step 2: Clean Out Your Pantry and Restock Smartly

One of the best ways to commit to a no-carb, no-sugar diet is by creating an environment that supports your success. Think of your kitchen as your ally—it's much easier to stay on track when your pantry and fridge are filled with nourishing options. This step is about removing temptations, stocking healthier alternatives, and making sure your kitchen is ready to fuel your new lifestyle.

Declutter Your Kitchen

The first move in this process is to thoroughly declutter your pantry, fridge, and freezer. Get rid of the foods that conflict with your no-carb, no-sugar goals. This includes obvious culprits as well as those sneaky items hiding sugar or carbs in unexpected forms.

What to remove:

- ***Packaged carbs***: Bread, pasta, crackers, cereals, granola, rice, tortillas, chips, and baked goods.
- ***Sugary items***: Candy bars, ice cream, chocolate spreads, syrups, soda, sweetened beverages, fruit juices, jams, and other sweetened condiments.
- ***Processed snacks***: Store-bought granola bars, muffins, cereal bars, snack cakes, and popcorn.
- ***High-carb pantry items***: Flour, cornstarch, bread crumbs, and premade seasoning mixes that include sugar.
- ***Hidden sugars***: Ketchup, barbecue sauce, salad dressings, marinades, yogurts, and even canned soups often contain added sugars.

Tip for success: Create a checklist, and as you go through each cabinet or drawer, mark off the items you're removing. This keeps the process organized and ensures nothing is overlooked.

Master the Art of Reading Labels

Once you start clearing out your kitchen, you'll quickly realize a lot of foods contain hidden sugars and carbs. That's why label reading is a crucial skill. Pay attention to both the nutrition facts panel and the ingredients list.

What to look for:

- Added sugars often sneak in under different names like glucose, sucrose, honey, agave, corn syrup, maltose, and molasses.
- High-carb ingredients such as wheat, oats, corn, and other grains.
- Net carbs (total carbs minus fiber) listed on the label—these are what impact your diet.

Pro Tip: If sugar is listed within the first three ingredients or if the product contains more than 5 grams of net carbs per serving, it's likely not suitable for your plan.

Restock with No-Carb, No-Sugar Essentials

Now comes the fun part—refilling your kitchen with foods that align with your goals! Make sure you have a variety of items on hand to keep your meals satisfying and interesting.

1. **Stock your pantry with**
     - Healthy fats like olive oil, avocado oil, and coconut oil.
     - Nuts and seeds (unsweetened and unprocessed), such as almonds, sunflower seeds, and chia seeds.
     - Broth or stock (look for no-sugar-added options).
     - Low-carb condiments like mustard, apple cider vinegar, hot sauce, and sugar-free salsa.

2. **Fill your fridge with:**
    - Protein-packed options like eggs, chicken, turkey, ground beef, and fish (salmon, tuna, or cod).
    - Non-starchy vegetables like spinach, kale, broccoli, cauliflower, zucchini, asparagus, and bell peppers.
    - Healthy snacks like cheese sticks, hard-boiled eggs, and no-sugar-added deli meats.
    - Full-fat dairy such as cream cheese, sour cream, and heavy whipping cream (in moderation).

Keep some freezer essentials:

- Frozen vegetables (without added sauces or sugars) for quick meals.
- Individually frozen proteins like shrimp, chicken breasts, or fish fillets.
- Frozen berries (used sparingly, as they're naturally low in sugar).

3. **Prepare Your Kitchen for Success**

Once your kitchen is decluttered and restocked, take a few extra steps to make it diet-friendly and easy to use—even on the busiest days.

- ***Organize for visibility***: Keep your go-to no-carb, no-sugar staples front and center. Use

clear storage containers for easy access to nuts, seeds, or pre-chopped veggies.
- *Create snack zones*: Dedicate a section of the fridge or shelves to ready-to-eat, no-carb snacks for those grab-and-go moments.
- *Batch prep basics*: Boil eggs, portion out cheese sticks, or sauté a big batch of veggies ahead of time so there's always something ready to eat.

4. **Strategize for Treats and On-the-Go**

Being prepared isn't just for eating at home—it's also important to plan for busy days or social events.

- *No-carb treats*: There are now no-sugar-added chocolates and keto-friendly snacks on the market that can help curb cravings.
- *Travel-proof items*: Stock up on portable snacks like beef jerky (no added sugar), nut butter packets, and low-carb protein bars.
- *Eating out*: Keep a mental list of low-carb-friendly takeout or restaurant meals to rely on when you're too busy to cook.

Cleaning out your pantry and restocking it sets the stage for success. When your kitchen aligns with your goals, it's easier to stick to your no-carb, no-sugar diet—even when things get hectic. Plus, knowing you've put in this effort to create a supportive environment is incredibly motivating! Stay organized, keep your favorite staples on hand, and enjoy the satisfaction of building a kitchen that works for your health.

Step 3: Make Smart Grocery Choices

A well-thought-out plan helps you avoid last-minute decisions that could lead to unhealthy choices. It's all about crafting balanced meals, staying ahead of your busy schedule, and building in variety, so you never feel deprived. Here's how you can build your ideal diet plan:

Start with the Basics of Your Meal Plan

Each meal should prioritize the following three components for optimal nutrition and satisfaction:

- *Protein*: Essential for maintaining energy levels, building muscle, and keeping hunger at bay. Go for options like eggs, chicken, turkey, fish, lean beef, and plant-based proteins if preferred.
- *Healthy Fats*: These provide lasting fullness and are vital for absorbing vitamins. Include avocados, nuts, seeds, olive oil, and fatty fish like salmon.
- *Non-Starchy Vegetables*: These are your source of essential vitamins, minerals, and fiber. Focus on spinach, cauliflower, zucchini, broccoli, asparagus, and bell peppers.

When building your meals, aim for a protein + a fat + a vegetable as your foundation. For example, grilled chicken with a side of roasted zucchini and a drizzle of olive oil.

Plan Your Day Strategically

To stay on track with a no-carb, no-sugar diet, divide your day into easy, balanced meals and snacks:

Breakfast

Kickstart your morning with protein and healthy fats to energize your day while avoiding carbs.

Examples include:

- Scrambled eggs with spinach and avocado slices.
- A small omelette with mushrooms, cheese, and a side of sautéed kale.
- A chia seed "pudding" made with unsweetened almond milk and topped with a sprinkle of unsweetened coconut flakes.

Lunch

Focus on meals you can pack for work or prepare quickly at home.

Examples include:

- Grilled chicken salad with mixed greens, cucumber, olives, and a lemon-olive oil dressing.

- Ground turkey or beef lettuce wraps with guacamole.
- Baked salmon with steamed broccoli and a drizzle of garlic butter.

Dinner

Keep it simple but satisfying after a long day.

Examples include:

- Steak with a side of roasted Brussels sprouts and cauliflower mash.
- Tuna salad served on fresh Romaine lettuce leaves instead of bread.
- Baked zucchini stuffed with ground turkey, tomatoes, and melted cheese.

Snacks

Stay fueled during the day with low-carb, no-sugar snacks that are portable and quick to eat.

Examples include:

- Cheese sticks paired with a few olives.
- A handful of macadamia nuts or walnuts.
- No-sugar-added beef jerky.

Prevent Boredom with Variety

Eating the same meals every day can lead to burnout. Keep things exciting by introducing new flavors, cooking techniques, and ingredient combinations.

- Try cooking vegetables in different ways—roast them with spices, steam them, or toss them in a stir-fry.
- Experiment with seasoning blends, such as Cajun, Italian, or garlic and herb.
- Rotate your proteins—swap chicken for shrimp, or try out lamb and bison for variety.
- Incorporate keto-friendly sauces or dressings, like pesto, garlic aioli, or a creamy herb dip.

Tip: Pinterest, cookbooks, and low-carb recipe websites can be a treasure trove of ideas if you're feeling uninspired.

Invest in Meal Prepping and Batch Cooking

For busy schedules, batch cooking and meal prepping can save time while keeping you on track. Dedicate an hour or two each week to prepare key ingredients you can mix and match.

- *Proteins*: Grill or bake chicken breasts, boil eggs, or brown ground turkey to have ready for meals.
- *Veggies*: Chop and roast a variety of vegetables that can be reheated all week long.

- ***Snacks***: Portion out nuts, jerky, or even homemade snacks like celery sticks with almond butter in advance.
- ***Sauces/Dressings***: Make a batch of sugar-free marinara, cheese sauce, or vinaigrette to dress up your meals quickly.

Tip: Store prepped ingredients in clear containers so you can easily see what's available.

Adjust Your Plan for Your Lifestyle

Whether you're a working mom, a student, or balancing multiple roles, your diet should fit neatly into your life. It's okay to adapt where needed—don't aim for perfection, just consistency.

- ***For busy mornings***: Opt for meals you can prepare the night before, like a pre-made omelette or boiled eggs.
- ***Flexible lunches***: Keep a stash of reliable low-carb options at work, like tuna cans, avocado, or pre-packed salads.
- ***Cook once, eat twice***: Double portions of dinner and pack leftovers for lunch the next day.
- ***Plan for emergencies***: Have a mental list of nearby restaurants or grocery store items you can grab when life throws a curveball.

Creating a no-carb, no-sugar diet plan can be simple. Stay organized, prep ahead, and include a variety of tasty, nourishing foods. By tailoring your plan to your lifestyle, you set yourself up for success—whether you have a busy schedule or need easy, reliable solutions.

Step 4: Track Your Progress

Charting your progress is an essential part of staying motivated and seeing how your commitment is paying off over time. Keeping track of changes in your weight, energy levels, mood, and how your body feels can give you a clearer picture of your overall progress.

Regular weigh-ins, weekly progress photos, or even measurements of your waist, hips, or other areas can help you stay on track and visualize your results.

Don't forget to celebrate non-scale victories, such as improved sleep quality, reduced cravings, higher energy, or feeling more confident in your daily activities—these wins are just as meaningful as the numbers on the scale.

Keeping a food diary or using an app to log your meals, workouts, and habits can help you spot patterns, identify what works best for you, and fine-tune your routine to suit your lifestyle better. Reflecting on your progress and small wins regularly can keep you inspired and focused on your long-term goals.

Step 5: Reach Out for Support

A busy lifestyle demands a sustainable and realistic plan, and consulting a healthcare professional or dietitian can make all the difference in achieving your health goals. These experts can help tailor your diet to suit your unique needs, whether you're managing specific health concerns like PCOS, diabetes, or high blood pressure, or simply aiming for better overall wellness.

They bring a wealth of knowledge and experience to address nutritional gaps, design meal plans that align with your preferences, and ensure you're meeting your body's requirements. Additionally, as your body changes over time—whether due to age, activity levels, or other factors—they can help you make necessary adjustments to your diet.

This personalized guidance not only keeps you safe but also makes it easier to stay consistent and maintain your progress in the long term. Seeking expert advice is a proactive step toward building healthier habits that truly last.

This guide proves that a no-carb, no-sugar diet can work for even the busiest women. With thoughtful preparation, small steps, and flexibility, you can achieve your goals with confidence and ease.

Foods to Eat in a No-Carb, No-Sugar Diet

A no-carb, no-sugar diet focuses on whole, unprocessed foods that are naturally low in carbohydrates and free from added sugars. Here's a comprehensive list, organized by food categories, to guide your choices:

Proteins

Protein is essential for building and repairing tissues, supporting metabolism, and keeping you full. Choose high-quality, unprocessed sources:

- *Meats*: Beef, pork, lamb, chicken, turkey, and game meats. Opt for fresh cuts like steaks, roasts, or ground options without added marinades or fillers.
- *Fish and Seafood*: Salmon, cod, mackerel, tuna, shrimp, crab, scallops, and mussels. These provide high-quality protein and healthy omega-3 fats.
- *Eggs*: Versatile and low in carbs, eggs are a perfect choice for any meal. Hard-boil them for an easy snack or incorporate them into various dishes.

Non-Starchy Vegetables

Non-starchy vegetables are low in carbs and rich in fiber, vitamins, and minerals. These are ideal for filling your plate:

- *Leafy Greens*: Spinach, kale, romaine, arugula, and Swiss chard. Use these as the base for salads or as a side dish.

- ***Cruciferous Vegetables***: Cauliflower, broccoli, Brussels sprouts, and cabbage. These are great for roasting or steaming.
- ***Zucchini and Summer Squash***: Spiralize for low-carb pasta or sauté in olive oil for a quick side.
- ***Bell Peppers***: Perfect for adding crunch and color to your meals.
- ***Mushrooms***: Low in carbs and great for sautéing or grilling.
- ***Cucumbers and Celery***: Hydrating and perfect as snacks or in salads.

Dairy (Unsweetened and Full-Fat)

Dairy provides calcium, protein, and healthy fats, but always choose unsweetened options to avoid hidden sugars:

- ***Cheese***: Cheddar, mozzarella, parmesan, gouda, cream cheese, and goat cheese are ideal choices.
- ***Greek Yogurt***: Stick to plain, full-fat versions with no added sugars.
- ***Heavy Cream and Unsweetened Creamer***: Use for coffee or recipes requiring a creamy texture.
- ***Butter or Ghee***: Rich in flavor and an excellent cooking fat for a no-carb diet.

Healthy Fats

Healthy fats are a vital energy source and help keep you satiated. Pick these foods to incorporate essential fats into your meals:

- *Avocados*: Excellent as a snack, in salads, or blended into smoothies.
- *Olive Oil*: Best for dressings, marinades, or low-temperature cooking.
- *Coconut Oil*: Useful for cooking, baking, or adding to coffee.
- *Nuts and Seeds*: Almonds, walnuts, pecans, macadamia nuts, chia seeds, flaxseeds, and sunflower seeds (unsweetened and in moderation).
- *Nut Butters*: Almond or macadamia nut butter without added sugar or oils.
- *Fatty Fish*: Salmon, sardines, and mackerel are both high in omega-3s and heart-healthy.

Pantry Staples

These items are perfect for cooking and baking while adhering to your diet:

- *Almond Flour and Coconut Flour*: For low-carb baking or breading.
- *Unsweetened Almond or Coconut Milk*: Use as a substitute for milk in recipes or beverages.

- ***Sugar-Free Condiments***: Mustard, vinegar, hot sauce, soy sauce, or coconut aminos (check labels for hidden sugars).
- ***Herbs and Spices***: Basil, oregano, thyme, cinnamon, turmeric, and cayenne pepper to flavor your meals.

Snacks

Keep these options on hand for when hunger strikes to avoid reaching for non-compliant foods:

- ***Hard-Boiled Eggs***: Prepared ahead of time for quick snacking.
- ***Olives***: A satisfying, salty option.
- ***Jerky***: Beef or turkey jerky without added sugar.
- ***Pork Rinds***: A crunchy, carb-free snack.

Drinks

Hydration is key while on this diet, and you can enjoy the following:

- ***Water***: Essential and can be flavored with lemon, lime, or cucumber slices.
- ***Herbal Tea***: Unsweetened and naturally caffeine-free options.
- ***Coffee or Tea***: Serve black or with a splash of heavy cream or unsweetened almond milk.
- ***Sparkling Water***: Plain or flavored versions with no added sugars.

By focusing on these food groups and avoiding anything processed or high in sugar, you can successfully stick to a no-carb, no-sugar diet while enjoying a variety of delicious and nutritious options

Foods to Avoid in a No-Carb, No-Sugar Diet

Sticking to a no-carb, no-sugar diet means cutting out foods that are high in carbohydrates and sugars. Below is a detailed list categorized for clarity, including specific examples and explanations.

1. **Grains and Grain-Based Products**

   These foods are high in carbohydrates and often spike blood sugar levels.

   - Bread (white, whole grain, rye, etc.)
   - Pasta (regular, whole wheat, gluten-free made from grains)
   - Rice (white, brown, wild, and other variants)
   - Cereal (both sugary and unsweetened varieties)
   - Tortillas (corn or flour-based)
   - Quinoa, Oats, Couscous

   Why avoid? Grains are carbohydrate-dense and can hinder compliance with a no-carb diet.

2. **Fruits**

   While fruits contain natural sugars, their carbohydrate content can still be too high for this diet.

   - Bananas
   - Mangoes
   - Grapes
   - Pineapples
   - Apples and Pears
   - Oranges and other sweet citrus fruits like mandarins

   Why avoid? Even though they're natural, the sugars in fruits contribute to carbohydrate intake.

3. **Certain Vegetables**

   Avoid starchy and high-carb veggies that can contribute significantly to carb intake.

   - Potatoes (white, red, sweet)
   - Corn
   - Peas
   - Carrots (in larger quantities)
   - Parsnips

   Why avoid? These vegetables are higher in starch, which converts to sugar during digestion.

4. **Dairy Products with Sugar or Carbs**

   Some dairy products contain added sugars or natural sugars like lactose.

   - Milk (whole, skim, and flavored varieties)
   - Flavored Yogurts (even if labeled "low-fat" or "low-sugar")
   - Ice Cream
   - Sweetened Dairy Drinks (like chocolate milk)

   Why avoid? Lactose (milk sugar) and added sugars increase your carb count. Stick to unsweetened, high-fat dairy.

5. **Sweetened and High-Sugar Beverages**

   These are loaded with sugar, even if marketed as healthy.

   - Sodas (regular and diet)
   - Fruit Juices (orange, apple, cranberry, etc.)
   - Sweetened Coffees and Teas (including frappuccinos and lattes)
   - Sports Drinks and flavored drinks like vitamin water
   - Alcoholic Beverages (beer, sweet wines, cocktails with sugary mixers)

   Why avoid? These drinks are some of the biggest culprits for hidden sugars and carbs.

6. **Processed and Packaged Foods**

   Most packaged or processed foods contain hidden sugars, starches, or preservatives with carbs.

   - Packaged Snack Bars (granola bars, protein bars)
   - Candy and Chocolates (even "sugar-free" often contain artificial sweeteners that affect blood sugar)
   - Chips, Crackers, Pretzels
   - Frozen Meals (like lasagna, pizza, or instant noodles)
   - Processed Meats (sausages, hot dogs with fillers, breaded chicken tenders)

   Why avoid? These foods often contain added ingredients like sugar, wheat, or corn syrup that are incompatible with this diet.

7. **Sugary Condiments and Sauces**

   Many condiments and dressings are filled with hidden sugars.

   - Ketchup
   - Barbecue Sauce
   - Sweetened Salad Dressings (like honey mustard or balsamic glaze)

- Marinades (often contain molasses, honey, or sugar)
- Sweetened Nut Butter (like regular peanut butter with added sugar)

Why avoid? These add unnecessary sugar and carbs to meals. Choose unsweetened or sugar-free options instead.

8. **Legumes and Beans**

While high in fiber, legumes are also high in carbs.

- Lentils
- Chickpeas (and products like hummus)
- Black Beans, Kidney Beans, Pinto Beans
- Soy Products (soy milk, soy-based snacks)

Why avoid? The carb content in legumes makes it difficult to fit into a strict no-carb guideline.

9. **Artificial or Hidden Sweeteners**

Some sweeteners can still impact carbs or trigger cravings.

- Honey, Agave Syrup, Maple Syrup
- Cane Sugar, Coconut Sugar
- Sugar Alcohols like Maltitol (common in sugar-free candies but can still impact blood sugar)

Why avoid? These may be marketed as "natural" or "low-sugar," but they still add carbs to your diet.

10. **Baked Goods and Desserts**

Virtually all traditional baked goods are off-limits.

- Cakes, Pies, Cookies
- Donuts, Muffins, Pastries
- Brownies and Cupcakes

Why avoid? These foods are typically made with processed sugars, grains, and other high-carb ingredients.

By eliminating these foods from your diet, you can stay on track and enjoy the benefits of a no-carb, no-sugar lifestyle. Replace them with low-carb staples like fresh vegetables, high-quality proteins, and healthy fats to maintain a satisfying and nutritious diet.

7-Day No Carbs and No Sugar Meal Plan

We have created a 7-day meal plan looking to follow a no-carb, no-sugar lifestyle. This sample meal plan includes easy and delicious recipes that are low in carbs and sugar while still providing all the essential nutrients your body needs.

Day 1

Breakfast

- Spinach & Cheese Omelette (2 large eggs, handful of spinach, 1 oz shredded cheddar cheese cooked in olive oil).
- Optional drink: Black coffee or unsweetened herbal tea.

AM Snack

10 Almonds (raw or roasted, unsalted).

Lunch

Grilled Lemon Herb Chicken (4 oz chicken breast marinated in olive oil, lemon juice, garlic, and herbs) with a side of sautéed zucchini (1 cup, cooked with garlic and olive oil).

PM Snack

- 1 Boiled Egg
- 2 celery sticks with 1 tbsp almond butter.

Dinner

Baked Salmon with Steamed Broccoli (4 oz salmon baked with olive oil, salt, pepper, and dill, served with 1 cup steamed broccoli).

Day 2

Breakfast

>Avocado Egg Cups (1 avocado halved and baked with an egg in each half; seasoned with salt and pepper).

AM Snack

>Small Handful of Brazil Nuts (5-6 pieces).

Lunch

>Grilled Steak Salad (4 oz grilled steak over mixed greens, cucumber slices, cherry tomatoes, and 1 tbsp olive oil as dressing).

PM Snack

- 1 String Cheese Stick
- 1 small cucumber sliced with a sprinkle of sea salt.

Dinner

Garlic-Butter Shrimp (5 oz shrimp cooked with olive oil, butter, and minced garlic) served with roasted asparagus (1 cup).

Day 3

Breakfast

Scrambled Eggs with Turkey Sausage (2 eggs scrambled with 2 oz turkey sausage and 1 tbsp olive oil).

AM Snack

1/4 Cup Pumpkin Seeds (raw or lightly roasted).

Lunch

Turkey Lettuce Wraps (3 large romaine leaves wrapped around 4 oz turkey breast, 1 tbsp mayo, and mustard).

PM Snack

- Hard-Boiled Egg
- A handful of snap peas.

Dinner

>Grilled Chicken Thighs (skin-on, 5 oz grilled with spices) served with steamed cauliflower rice (1 cup).

Day 4

Breakfast

>Vegetable Frittata (2 eggs whisked with 1/4 cup diced bell peppers, onions, and spinach, cooked in olive oil).

AM Snack

>10 Pecan (unsalted, raw, or roasted).

Lunch

>Grilled Trout with Roasted Brussels Sprouts (4 oz trout grilled and seasoned with olive oil and lemon, served with 1 cup roasted Brussels sprouts).

PM Snack

>1/4 Avocado with sea salt and red pepper flakes.

Dinner

>Zucchini Noodles with Pesto Shrimp (1 cup zucchini spirals sautéed in olive oil topped with grilled shrimp and 2 tbsp sugar-free pesto).

Day 5

Breakfast

Poached Eggs with Sliced Avocado (2 eggs and 1/2 avocado seasoned with sea salt and black pepper).

AM Snack

Small Handful of Walnuts.

Lunch

Herb-Roasted Chicken with Spinach Salad (4 oz roasted chicken breast served on 2 cups fresh spinach with olive oil drizzle).

PM Snack

1 Cup Cherry Tomatoes sprinkled lightly with sea salt.

Dinner

Pan-Seared Cod with Sautéed Kale (4 oz cod cooked in olive oil served with 1 cup kale sautéed with garlic).

Day 6

Breakfast

Egg Muffins (2 muffins made with eggs, sautéed mushrooms, diced bell peppers, and shredded cheddar cheese).

AM Snack

2 Celery Sticks with 2 tbsp guacamole.

Lunch

Grilled Lamb Chops (4 oz lamb chops served with roasted eggplant and zucchini seasoned with olive oil, garlic, and herbs).

PM Snack

1 Ounce Macadamia Nuts.

Dinner

Roasted Duck Breast with Cauliflower Mash (4 oz duck breast roasted with olive oil served with 1 cup mashed cauliflower).

Day 7

Breakfast

Stuffed Bell Peppers (1 bell pepper halved and baked with 2 eggs, salt, and pepper).

AM Snack

Small Handful of Cashews (10-12 pieces).

Lunch

> Tuna Salad on Romaine Leaves (4 oz tuna mixed with mayonnaise, diced celery, and salt, served on 3 large romaine leaves).

PM Snack

- 1 Baby Bell Cheese Wheel
- 1/2 cucumber sliced with a squeeze of lemon juice.

Dinner

> Grilled Pork Chops with Steamed Green Beans (5 oz pork chops grilled, served with 1 cup steamed green beans and a pat of butter).

This meal plan prioritizes variety, nutrient intake, and simplicity. Make sure to hydrate throughout the day and consult with a healthcare provider to confirm the diet aligns with your personal health needs.

Sample Recipes

To help you get started, here are some simple and nutritious recipes that align with this meal plan:

Spinach & Cheese Omelette Recipe

Ingredients:

- 2 large eggs
- A handful of fresh spinach (roughly 1 cup, loosely packed)
- 1 oz shredded cheddar cheese
- 1 tbsp olive oil for cooking
- Optional seasonings: salt, pepper, garlic powder (a pinch of each)
- Optional garnish: fresh parsley or chives, finely chopped

Instructions:

1. In a small mixing bowl, beat the eggs with a fork or whisk until well combined.
2. Heat olive oil in a non-stick pan over medium heat.
3. Add spinach to the pan and cook for 1-2 minutes, stirring occasionally until it starts to wilt.
4. Pour the beaten eggs into the pan, making sure they cover all of the spinach evenly.
5. Sprinkle shredded cheddar cheese on top of the eggs and season with salt, pepper, and garlic powder if desired.
6. Cook for about 3-4 minutes or until the edges start to crisp up and turn golden brown.

7. Using a spatula, carefully fold one side of the omelette over the other, creating a half-moon shape.
8. Cook for an additional 1-2 minutes or until the cheese is fully melted and the eggs are cooked through.
9. Serve hot with a sprinkle of fresh parsley or chives on top for added flavor if desired.

Grilled Lemon Herb Chicken with Sautéed Zucchini

Ingredients:

For the Chicken:

- 4 oz chicken breast
- 2 tbsp olive oil (divided)
- 2 tbsp fresh lemon juice (about half a lemon)
- 2 garlic cloves, minced
- 1 tsp mixed dried herbs (or a combination of thyme, rosemary, and oregano)
- Optional seasonings: salt and black pepper to taste
- Optional garnish: chopped fresh parsley or a lemon wedge

For the Zucchini:

- 1 medium zucchini (about 1 cup when sliced)
- 1 tbsp olive oil
- 1 garlic clove, minced
- Optional seasonings: salt, pepper, and a pinch of red chili flakes for a hint of heat

Instructions:

1. Marinate the Chicken: In a small bowl, mix 1 tablespoon olive oil, lemon juice, minced garlic, and dried herbs. Add salt and black pepper if desired. Place the chicken in a shallow dish or ziplock bag, pour the

marinade over, and ensure it's evenly coated. Marinate for at least 30 minutes or overnight in the fridge.

2. Heat the Grill or Skillet: Preheat your grill to medium-high heat (375-400°F) or heat a skillet over medium-high heat.
3. Grill the Chicken: Remove chicken from the marinade and discard the rest. Cook on the grill or skillet for 6-7 minutes per side, until the internal temperature reaches 165°F and juices run clear.
4. Cook the Zucchini: Slice zucchini into rounds or strips. In a pan, heat olive oil over medium heat. Add minced garlic and stir for 30 seconds until fragrant. Add zucchini and sauté for 5-6 minutes until tender. Season with salt, pepper, and chili flakes if desired.
5. Serve: Serve the chicken and zucchini hot, either together or side by side.

Avocado Egg Cups Recipe

Ingredients:

- 1 ripe avocado
- 2 large eggs
- Salt, to taste
- Freshly ground black pepper, to taste
- Optional seasonings or garnishes:
- Red pepper flakes or hot sauce for a spicy kick
- Fresh herbs like parsley, cilantro, or chives, finely chopped
- Shredded cheese (cheddar, Parmesan, or mozzarella)

Instructions:

1. Prep the Ingredients: Set the oven to 375°F (190°C) and allow it to preheat. Rinse the avocado, slice it in half, and take out the pit. Remove a small portion from the center of each half to make space for the egg. Keep the removed avocado aside to use as a topping or enjoy as a snack later.
2. Stabilize the Avocado Halves: Place the avocado halves in a baking dish or on a rimmed baking sheet. Use crumpled foil or an oven-safe ramekin to nestle them so they don't tip over during baking.
3. Add the Eggs: Carefully crack an egg into each avocado half. If your avocado is small, you may need to pour out a little egg white to avoid overflow.

Sprinkle the tops with salt and freshly ground black pepper for seasoning.
4. Bake the Avocado Egg Cups: Place the baking dish or sheet in the oven and bake for 15-20 minutes, or until the egg whites are set and the yolks are cooked to your liking. For a runny yolk, check around the 15-minute mark; for firmer yolks, leave it closer to 20.
5. Add Optional Toppings: Once done, remove the avocado egg cups from the oven. Add any desired toppings, such as a sprinkle of shredded cheese, fresh herbs, or a dash of hot sauce.
6. Serve: Serve the avocado egg cups warm, either on their own or with a simple side like a small green salad or crispy bacon for extra protein.

Grilled Steak Salad

Ingredients:

- 4 oz steak
- 2 cups mixed greens
- 1/2 cucumber, sliced
- 1/2 cup cherry tomatoes, halved
- 1 tbsp olive oil (for dressing)
- Salt and pepper to taste
- Optional: 1 tbsp balsamic vinegar, crumbled feta, or fresh herbs

Instructions:

1. Prepare the Steak: Season the steak with salt and pepper to your liking. Heat a grill or grill pan over medium-high heat and cook the steak for about 4-5 minutes on each side, or until desired level of doneness is reached. Let rest for 5 minutes before slicing.
2. Assemble Salad: In a large bowl, combine mixed greens, sliced cucumber, and halved cherry tomatoes.
3. Make Dressing: Whisk together olive oil, balsamic vinegar (if using), salt, and pepper in a small bowl.
4. Add Steak Slices: Slice the rested steak against the grain into thin strips and add to the salad.
5. Toss Everything Together: Pour dressing over the salad and steak slices, then toss to evenly coat all ingredients.

6. Optional: Add Additional Toppings: If desired, top with crumbled feta or fresh herbs for extra flavor and texture.
7. Serve: Divide the grilled steak salad onto plates and serve immediately.

Scrambled Eggs with Turkey Sausage

Ingredients:

- 2 large eggs
- 2 oz turkey sausage, crumbled
- 1 tbsp olive oil
- Salt and pepper to taste
- Optional garnishes: fresh herbs (like parsley or chives) or shredded cheese

Instructions:

1. Cook Sausage: Heat a non-stick pan over medium-high heat and add crumbled turkey sausage. Cook for about 5-6 minutes, stirring occasionally, until browned and cooked through.
2. Scramble Eggs: In a separate bowl, crack the eggs and whisk together with salt and pepper.
3. Add Eggs to Pan: Make a well in the center of the sausage in the pan, then pour the beaten eggs into it.
4. Continuously Scramble Eggs: Using a spatula or wooden spoon, continuously stir and fold the eggs as they cook for about 2-3 minutes, until fluffy and no longer runny.
5. Garnish and Serve: Sprinkle with fresh herbs or shredded cheese (if desired) and serve hot on a plate or in a bowl.

Turkey Lettuce Wraps

Ingredients:

- 3 large romaine leaves
- 4 oz turkey breast (sliced)
- 1 tbsp mayonnaise
- Mustard, to taste
- Optional additions: sliced tomatoes, shredded cheese, or avocado slices

Instructions:

1. Wash and Prep Lettuce: Carefully wash and dry the romaine leaves, then lay them flat on a cutting board.
2. Spread Mayonnaise: Spread mayonnaise evenly over each lettuce leaf, leaving about an inch of space around the edges.
3. Add Turkey Slices: Place sliced turkey breast on top of the mayonnaise in a single layer.
4. Add Mustard and Optional Toppings: Drizzle mustard over the turkey slices and add any desired toppings such as sliced tomatoes, shredded cheese, or avocado slices.
5. Roll Up Wraps: Starting at one end, tightly roll up each lettuce wrap until all ingredients are securely tucked inside.

6. Cut and Serve: Use a sharp knife to cut each wrap in half, then serve immediately or pack for a delicious and healthy on-the-go meal.

Grilled Chicken Thighs with Steamed Cauliflower Rice

Ingredients:

- 5 oz skin-on chicken thighs
- Spices for seasoning (e.g., paprika, garlic powder, salt, and pepper)
- 1 cup cauliflower rice
- Optional garnishes: fresh parsley, lemon wedges, or a drizzle of olive oil

Instructions:

1. Season and Grill the Chicken
2. Rub the chicken thighs with spices of your choice.
3. Grill over medium heat, skin-side down first, for 5-6 minutes per side until golden and cooked through (internal temp 165°F).
4. Steam the Cauliflower Rice: Place cauliflower rice in a steamer or microwave with a splash of water. Steam for 3-4 minutes until tender.
5. Serve: Plate the grilled chicken with cauliflower rice. Garnish with parsley or a squeeze of lemon if desired.

Vegetable Frittata

Ingredients:

- 2 large eggs
- 1/4 cup diced bell peppers
- 1/4 cup diced onions
- 1/4 cup chopped spinach
- 1 tbsp olive oil
- Salt and pepper to taste
- Optional toppings: shredded cheese or fresh herbs

Instructions:

1. Prepare the Vegetables: In a small skillet, heat olive oil over medium heat. Add diced peppers and onions and sauté for 2-3 minutes until softened.
2. Whisk Eggs: In a mixing bowl, whisk together eggs, chopped spinach, salt, and pepper.
3. Add Eggs to Skillet: Pour egg mixture into the skillet with vegetables, making sure they are evenly distributed.
4. Cook Frittata: Cover the skillet and let cook on medium-low heat for about 5 minutes until the edges appear set.
5. Optional Toppings: If desired, sprinkle shredded cheese or fresh herbs over the frittata before covering to cook.

6. Finish Cooking and Serve: Remove cover and continue cooking for another 2-3 minutes until the top is set and cooked through. Slide frittata onto a plate and serve hot. Optional: garnish with fresh herbs or a drizzle of olive oil on top.

Grilled Trout with Roasted Brussels Sprouts

Ingredients:

- 2 trout fillets
- 1/4 cup olive oil
- 2 cloves garlic, minced
- 1 tsp dried thyme
- Salt and pepper to taste
- 1 lb Brussels sprouts, halved
- Additional herbs for seasoning (optional)

Instructions:

1. Marinate Trout: In a shallow dish, mix together olive oil, minced garlic, dried thyme, salt and pepper. Add trout fillets and coat well with the marinade. Let marinate in the fridge for at least 30 minutes.
2. Preheat Grill: Preheat grill to medium heat (350°F).
3. Prepare Brussels Sprouts: In a bowl, toss halved Brussels sprouts with olive oil and season with salt, pepper, and additional herbs if desired.
4. Grill Trout: Place marinated trout fillets on the preheated grill. Grill for 3-5 minutes on each side or until fish flakes easily with a fork.
5. Roast Brussels Sprouts: While the trout is cooking, place the seasoned Brussels sprouts onto a foil-lined baking sheet and roast in the oven for about 15 minutes at 375°F.

6. Serve: Once cooked, remove trout from grill and serve hot with roasted Brussels sprouts on the side. Optional: garnish with additional herbs for added flavor.

Zucchini Noodles with Pesto Shrimp

Ingredients:

- 4 zucchini, spiralized
- 1 lb shrimp, peeled and deveined
- 2 tbsp olive oil
- Salt and pepper to taste
- 1/2 cup pesto sauce
- Grated Parmesan cheese for topping (optional)

Instructions:

1. Prepare Zucchini Noodles: Using a spiralizer or vegetable peeler, create thin noodles out of the zucchini. Set aside.
2. Cook Shrimp: In a pan over medium heat, add olive oil and shrimp. Season with salt and pepper to taste. Cook for about 3 minutes on each side until shrimp is pink.
3. Add Noodles and Pesto: Once the shrimp is cooked, add in the zucchini noodles and pesto sauce. Toss everything together until well coated.
4. Serve: Once the noodles are tender (about 2-3 minutes), remove from heat and serve hot. Optional: top with grated Parmesan cheese for added flavor.

Poached Eggs with Sliced Avocado

Ingredients:

- 4 eggs
- 1 ripe avocado, sliced
- Salt and pepper to taste
- Toasted whole wheat bread (optional)

Instructions:

1. Poach Eggs: Fill a medium-sized pot with about 3 inches of water and bring to a simmer. Crack each egg into a small bowl or cup. Once the water is simmering, use a spoon to stir the water in one direction until it creates a whirlpool effect. Slowly pour each egg into the center of the whirlpool. Cook for about 3 minutes until whites are set but yolks are still runny.
2. Toast Bread (Optional): While the eggs are cooking, toast slices of whole wheat bread.
3. Assemble: Once the eggs are cooked, remove them from the pot with a slotted spoon and place on a paper towel to drain any excess water. Season with salt and pepper to taste.
4. Serve: Place sliced avocado on top of each slice of toast (if using) and then add one poached egg on top. Optional: garnish with additional seasoning or herbs for added flavor.

Herb-Roasted Chicken with Spinach Salad

Ingredients:

- 4 boneless, skinless chicken breasts
- 2 tablespoons olive oil
- 1 teaspoon dried thyme
- 1 teaspoon dried rosemary
- Salt and pepper to taste
- 6 cups baby spinach leaves
- 1/4 cup sliced almonds
- 1/4 cup dried cranberries
- Balsamic vinaigrette dressing (optional)

Instructions:

1. Preheat Oven: Preheat your oven to 375 degrees Fahrenheit.
2. Prepare Chicken: Combine olive oil, thyme, rosemary, salt, and pepper in a small bowl. Use a brush to evenly coat both sides of the chicken breasts with the mixture.
3. Roast Chicken: Place the chicken breasts on a baking sheet and roast for 25-30 minutes, until they reach an internal temperature of 165 degrees Fahrenheit.
4. Prepare Salad: While the chicken is roasting, prepare your salad by combining baby spinach leaves, sliced almonds, and dried cranberries in a large bowl.

5. Add Dressing (Optional): If desired, drizzle balsamic vinaigrette dressing over the salad and toss to coat evenly.
6. Serve: Once the chicken is fully cooked, remove it from the oven and let it rest for a few minutes before slicing. Serve with the prepared spinach salad on the side.

Pan-Seared Cod with Sautéed Kale

Ingredients:

- 4 cod fillets
- 2 tablespoons olive oil
- 1 teaspoon garlic powder
- Salt and pepper to taste
- 6 cups chopped kale leaves
- 2 cloves of garlic, minced
- 1 tablespoon butter (or olive oil for a healthier option)

Instructions:

1. Season Cod: Season both sides of the cod fillets with garlic powder, salt, and pepper.
2. Heat Oil: Heat olive oil in a large skillet over medium-high heat.
3. Add Cod: Carefully place the seasoned cod fillets into the hot oil and cook for about 5 minutes on each side, or until they are fully cooked and flaky.
4. Sauté Kale: In a separate skillet, melt the butter (or heat olive oil) over medium-high heat. Add minced garlic and cook for about 1 minute.
5. Add Kale: Add chopped kale to the skillet with the garlic and sauté for about 3-4 minutes, until it is wilted and slightly crispy.

6. Serve: Plate the cod fillets with a serving of sautéed kale on the side. Garnish with additional salt and pepper if desired.

Conclusion

Thank you for completing this guide on adopting a no-carbs, no-sugar diet. By dedicating your time and attention, you've taken a meaningful step toward taking control of your health and well-being. Balancing a busy life with personal goals can be challenging, but armed with the strategies and insights provided in this guide, you now have the tools to make healthier choices that align with your demands.

This diet is about far more than just numbers on a scale. It's about reshaping the way you approach food, energy, and your overall lifestyle. Cutting out carbs and sugar helps stabilize your blood sugar levels, reduce cravings, and provide a steady energy source from wholesome proteins and fats. These changes can help you feel more alert, improve moods, and enhance your focus. No longer relying on bursts of energy from quick fixes like sugary snacks can leave you feeling like you're back in control of your day.

This is not a rigid process, nor does it have to be overwhelming. The key is starting with small, consistent habits. Maybe it's as simple as prepping meals on Sundays, swapping out bread for lettuce wraps, or carrying high-protein snacks to avoid unhealthy temptations. With each small adjustment, you're moving closer to a lifestyle that feels natural. Trust in the process and be kind to yourself along the way. Missteps might happen, but every decision to try again keeps you on the right path.

One of the strengths of this approach is its flexibility. With planning and preparation, you can fit this lifestyle into your busy schedule without unnecessary stress. Simple meal plans, easy recipes, and handy snacks make it easier to stick with your goals. This isn't about deprivation—it's about discovering meals that nourish and satisfy you while fitting seamlessly into your life. You are creating habits, not following temporary fixes, and those habits will support long-term success.

Take a moment to acknowledge your achievements outside of the scale. Maybe you're waking up with more energy, experiencing fewer cravings during the day, or noticing mental clarity that wasn't there before. Each of these victories is proof that you're making progress toward a stronger, healthier version of yourself. Celebrate these wins—they are milestones that reflect your hard work and commitment.

You're on a unique and personal health journey. This path is about you prioritizing your well-being amidst life's many demands. By committing to this lifestyle, you aren't just choosing to lose weight or gain better health; you're actively creating balance, resilience, and the ability to thrive. This process is yours to shape, adapt, and evolve as you grow.

Thank you again for dedicating yourself to this guide and for focusing on your health. Every step forward, no matter how small, reinforces your strength and determination. Continue believing in your ability to make these changes and trust that they'll empower you in the long run. Stay consistent, stay persistent, and know you're capable of achieving a healthier, more vibrant life—one choice at a time. You've got this.

FAQs

How can I start a no-carb, no-sugar diet with a busy schedule?

Start by dedicating 1-2 hours on weekends to meal prep. Batch-cook proteins, chop vegetables, and portion snacks for the week. Keep grab-and-go options like boiled eggs, cheese sticks, and nuts handy. Start with one no-carb, no-sugar meal a day and gradually increase. This makes the transition easier and less overwhelming.

What should I do if I experience cravings for carbs or sugar?

Cravings often come from habits or blood sugar changes. Fight them by eating balanced meals with protein, healthy fats, and fiber to stay full longer. Stay hydrated, as dehydration can feel like hunger. Keep low-sugar, low-carb snacks like dark chocolate (85%+), unsweetened whipped cream with berries, or roasted nuts on hand. Distract yourself with a walk or deep breathing until the craving fades.

How can I eat out or attend social events while staying on track?

When eating out, choose grilled meats, salads, or roasted vegetables. Ask for dressings or sauces on the side, and skip bread baskets or sugary drinks. For social events, eat a small meal beforehand and bring a dish like a veggie platter or meat skewers to ensure you have options.

What snacks can I keep on hand for busy days?

Quick snacks include boiled eggs, cheese cubes, celery sticks with almond butter, deli meat wrapped in lettuce, or a handful of nuts. Keep them in your bag, car, or desk to avoid high-carb options when hunger hits. Prepping these ahead of time saves stress during busy moments.

Will cutting carbs and sugar affect my energy levels?

At first, you may experience the "keto flu," with low energy as your body switches to burning fat instead of carbs. This typically lasts a few days. Stay hydrated, add a pinch of salt to water for electrolytes, and focus on meals with healthy fats and protein. Once adjusted, most people report steady, sustained energy.

Can I still treat myself while following this diet?

Yes! Try no-carb, no-sugar treats like fat bombs with unsweetened cocoa and coconut oil, or berries with whipped cream in moderation. Roasted nuts or pork rinds can also satisfy crunchy snack cravings. Treating yourself doesn't have to break your diet—there are plenty of delicious, compliant options.

How do I balance this diet with family meals or feeding kids?

Serve dishes everyone will enjoy, like grilled chicken, sautéed veggies, or lettuce wrap tacos. Add sides like rice or bread for those not following your diet. By using wholesome ingredients, you'll create nutritious meals that suit everyone while meeting your needs.

References and Helpful Links

Ld, L. S. M. R. (2024, March 1). What is a Zero-Carb diet, and what foods can you eat? Healthline.
https://www.healthline.com/nutrition/no-carb-diet

HealthMatch staff & HealthMatch Pty Ltd. (2022, March 6). What level of weight loss can you get on keto? Learn benefits and risks. HealthMatch.
https://healthmatch.io/weight-management/how-much-weight-can-you-lose-on-keto#:~:text=If%20a%20person%20follows%20the,around%20one%20pound%20per%20week

No sugar, no carbs meal ideas. (n.d.). Pinterest.
https://www.pinterest.com/initialthisthat/no-sugar-no-carbs-meal-ideas/

Johnson, J. (2019, December 13). What to know about no-sugar diets.
https://www.medicalnewstoday.com/articles/319991

What is the No Sugar, No Carb Diet? - Dr. Robert Kiltz. (2023, December 15). Dr. Robert Kiltz.
https://www.doctorkiltz.com/no-sugar-no-carb-diet/

Ld, L. S. M. R. (2024, March 1). What is a Zero-Carb diet, and what foods can you eat? Healthline.
https://www.healthline.com/nutrition/no-carb-diet

www.ingramcontent.com/pod-product-compliance
Lightning Source LLC
LaVergne TN
LVHW012031060526
838201LV00061B/4559